CONTENTS

◇ **PERSONALIZATION PAGE** — 1
◇ **PARENT(S) / GUARDIANS INFORMATION** — 2
◇ **EXTENDED MEDICAL INFORMATION** — 3-6
◇ **FAMILY MEDICAL HISTORY** — 7-8
◇ **INSURANCE DETAILS** — 9-10
◇ **IMMUNIZATION RECORD** — 11-23
◇ **TREATMENT HISTORY-MEDICATION** — 24-41
◇ **SYMPTOM TRACKER** — 42-61
◇ **TREATMENT HISTORY - VISITS** — 62-86
◇ **GROWTH / WEIGHT LOG** — 87-90
◇ **TEETH CHARTS** — 91
◇ **TOOTH RECORD** — 92
◇ **NOTES SECTION** — 93-102

THIS BOOK BELONGS TO

NAME_____GENDER_____

DATE OF BIRTH_____PLACE OF BIRTH_____

BIRTH WEIGHT_____BIRTH LENGTH_____

ADDRESS_____

_____

EYE COLOR_____SKIN COLOR_____

BLOOD GROUP_____ORGAN DONOR?   YES ☐   NO ☐

MEDICAL CONDITIONS_____

_____

ALLERGIES_____

EMERGENCY CONTACT 1

NAME_____

RELATIONSHIP_____

CONTACT NUMBER_____

ADDRESS_____

_____

COMMENTS_____

_____

EMERGENCY CONTACT 2

NAME_____

RELATIONSHIP_____

CONTACT NUMBER_____

ADDRESS_____

_____

COMMENTS_____

_____

PARENTS / GUARDIANS

NAME_____**GENDER**_____

DATE OF BIRTH_____**PLACE OF BIRTH**_____

ADDRESS_____

_____

BLOOD GROUP_____**ORGAN DONOR?**   YES ☐   NO ☐

MEDICAL CONDITIONS_____

_____

ALLERGIES_____

_____

NAME_____**GENDER**_____

DATE OF BIRTH_____**PLACE OF BIRTH**_____

ADDRESS_____

_____

BLOOD GROUP_____**ORGAN DONOR?**   YES ☐   NO ☐

MEDICAL CONDITIONS_____

_____

ALLERGIES_____

_____

COMMENTS

_____

_____

_____

_____

_____

_____

_____

EXTENDED MEDICAL INFORMATION

EXTENDED MEDICAL INFORMATION

EXTENDED MEDICAL INFORMATION

EXTENDED MEDICAL INFORMATION

FAMILY MEDICAL HISTORY

FATHER / PATERNAL GRANDPARENTS	YES	NO	COMMENTS
High Blood Pressure			
High Cholesterol			
Stroke			
Glaucoma			
Diabetes			
Epilepsy			
Asthma			
Allergies			
Hearing Loss			
Cancer (type)			
Kidney Problems			
Alcohol Misuse			
Drug Misuse			
Obesity			

FAMILY MEDICAL HISTORY

MOTHER / PATERNAL GRANDPARENTS	YES	NO	COMMENTS
High Blood Pressure			
High Cholesterol			
Stroke			
Glaucoma			
Diabetes			
Epilepsy			
Asthma			
Allergies			
Hearing Loss			
Cancer (type)			
Kidney Problems			
Alcohol Misuse			
Drug Misuse			
Obesity			

INSURANCE DETAILS

COMPANY _____

POLICY DETAILS _____

COVER DETAILS _____

ADDRESS _____

_____

_____

CONTACT NO: _____

EMAIL _____

WEBSITE _____

HEALTH CARE DETAILS

PEDIATRICIAN DETAILS

NAME: _____

ADDRESS: _____

_____

PHONE NUMBER: _____

DENTIST

NAME: _____

ADDRESS: _____

_____

PHONE NUMBER: _____

SPECIALIST

NAME: _____

ADDRESS: _____

_____

PHONE NUMBER: _____

INSURANCE DETAILS

COMPANY _____

POLICY DETAILS _____

COVER DETAILS _____

ADDRESS _____

_____

_____

CONTACT NO: _____

EMAIL _____

WEBSITE _____

HEALTH CARE DETAILS

PEDIATRICIAN DETAILS
NAME: _____
ADDRESS: _____
_____
PHONE NUMBER: _____

DENTIST
NAME: _____
ADDRESS: _____
_____
PHONE NUMBER: _____

SPECIALIST
NAME: _____
ADDRESS: _____
_____
PHONE NUMBER: _____

IMMUNIZATION RECORD

Vaccine:

Date administered:

Next Dose date:

Administered by:

Vaccine:

Date administered:

Next Dose date:

Administered by:

Vaccine:

Date administered:

Next Dose date:

Administered by:

Vaccine:

Date administered:

Next Dose date:

Administered by:

Vaccine:

Date administered:

Next Dose date:

Administered by:

Vaccine:

Date administered:

Next Dose date:

Administered by:

IMMUNIZATION RECORD

Vaccine:

Date administered:

Next Dose date:

Administered by:

Vaccine:

Date administered:

Next Dose date:

Administered by:

Vaccine:

Date administered:

Next Dose date:

Administered by:

Vaccine:

Date administered:

Next Dose date:

Administered by:

Vaccine:

Date administered:

Next Dose date:

Administered by:

Vaccine:

Date administered:

Next Dose date:

Administered by:

IMMUNIZATION RECORD

Vaccine:

Date administered:

Next Dose date:

Administered by:

Vaccine:

Date administered:

Next Dose date:

Administered by:

Vaccine:

Date administered:

Next Dose date:

Administered by:

Vaccine:

Date administered:

Next Dose date:

Administered by:

Vaccine:

Date administered:

Next Dose date:

Administered by:

Vaccine:

Date administered:

Next Dose date:

Administered by:

IMMUNIZATION RECORD

Vaccine:

Date administered:

Next Dose date:

Administered by:

Vaccine:

Date administered:

Next Dose date:

Administered by:

Vaccine:

Date administered:

Next Dose date:

Administered by:

Vaccine:

Date administered:

Next Dose date:

Administered by:

Vaccine:

Date administered:

Next Dose date:

Administered by:

Vaccine:

Date administered:

Next Dose date:

Administered by:

IMMUNIZATION RECORD

Vaccine:

Date administered:

Next Dose date:

Administered by:

Vaccine:

Date administered:

Next Dose date:

Administered by:

Vaccine:

Date administered:

Next Dose date:

Administered by:

Vaccine:

Date administered:

Next Dose date:

Administered by:

Vaccine:

Date administered:

Next Dose date:

Administered by:

Vaccine:

Date administered:

Next Dose date:

Administered by:

IMMUNIZATION RECORD

Vaccine:

Date administered:

Next Dose date:

Administered by:

Vaccine:

Date administered:

Next Dose date:

Administered by:

Vaccine:

Date administered:

Next Dose date:

Administered by:

Vaccine:

Date administered:

Next Dose date:

Administered by:

Vaccine:

Date administered:

Next Dose date:

Administered by:

Vaccine:

Date administered:

Next Dose date:

Administered by:

IMMUNIZATION RECORD

Vaccine:

Date administered:

Next Dose date:

Administered by:

Vaccine:

Date administered:

Next Dose date:

Administered by:

Vaccine:

Date administered:

Next Dose date:

Administered by:

Vaccine:

Date administered:

Next Dose date:

Administered by:

Vaccine:

Date administered:

Next Dose date:

Administered by:

Vaccine:

Date administered:

Next Dose date:

Administered by:

IMMUNIZATION RECORD

Vaccine:

Date administered:

Next Dose date:

Administered by:

Vaccine:

Date administered:

Next Dose date:

Administered by:

Vaccine:

Date administered:

Next Dose date:

Administered by:

Vaccine:

Date administered:

Next Dose date:

Administered by:

Vaccine:

Date administered:

Next Dose date:

Administered by:

Vaccine:

Date administered:

Next Dose date:

Administered by:

IMMUNIZATION RECORD

Vaccine:

Date administered:

Next Dose date:

Administered by:

Vaccine:

Date administered:

Next Dose date:

Administered by:

Vaccine:

Date administered:

Next Dose date:

Administered by:

Vaccine:

Date administered:

Next Dose date:

Administered by:

Vaccine:

Date administered:

Next Dose date:

Administered by:

Vaccine:

Date administered:

Next Dose date:

Administered by:

IMMUNIZATION RECORD

Vaccine:

Date administered:

Next Dose date:

Administered by:

Vaccine:

Date administered:

Next Dose date:

Administered by:

Vaccine:

Date administered:

Next Dose date:

Administered by:

Vaccine:

Date administered:

Next Dose date:

Administered by:

Vaccine:

Date administered:

Next Dose date:

Administered by:

Vaccine:

Date administered:

Next Dose date:

Administered by:

IMMUNIZATION RECORD

Vaccine:

Date administered:

Next Dose date:

Administered by:

Vaccine:

Date administered:

Next Dose date:

Administered by:

Vaccine:

Date administered:

Next Dose date:

Administered by:

Vaccine:

Date administered:

Next Dose date:

Administered by:

Vaccine:

Date administered:

Next Dose date:

Administered by:

Vaccine:

Date administered:

Next Dose date:

Administered by:

IMMUNIZATION RECORD

Vaccine:

Date administered:

Next Dose date:

Administered by:

Vaccine:

Date administered:

Next Dose date:

Administered by:

Vaccine:

Date administered:

Next Dose date:

Administered by:

Vaccine:

Date administered:

Next Dose date:

Administered by:

Vaccine:

Date administered:

Next Dose date:

Administered by:

Vaccine:

Date administered:

Next Dose date:

Administered by:

IMMUNIZATION RECORD

Vaccine:

Date administered:

Next Dose date:

Administered by:

Vaccine:

Date administered:

Next Dose date:

Administered by:

Vaccine:

Date administered:

Next Dose date:

Administered by:

Vaccine:

Date administered:

Next Dose date:

Administered by:

Vaccine:

Date administered:

Next Dose date:

Administered by:

Vaccine:

Date administered:

Next Dose date:

Administered by:

TREATMENT HISTORY - MEDICATION

MEDICATION NAME	DATE STARTED	START DOSE	DATE ENDED	END DOSE
FREQUENCY				
PRESCRIBING PHYSICIAN				
RESULT & COMMENTS				

MEDICATION NAME	DATE STARTED	START DOSE	DATE ENDED	END DOSE
FREQUENCY				
PRESCRIBING PHYSICIAN				
RESULT & COMMENTS				

MEDICATION NAME	DATE STARTED	START DOSE	DATE ENDED	END DOSE
FREQUENCY				
PRESCRIBING PHYSICIAN				
RESULT & COMMENTS				

TREATMENT HISTORY - MEDICATION

MEDICATION NAME	DATE STARTED	START DOSE	DATE ENDED	END DOSE
FREQUENCY				
PRESCRIBING PHYSICIAN				
RESULT & COMMENTS				

MEDICATION NAME	DATE STARTED	START DOSE	DATE ENDED	END DOSE
FREQUENCY				
PRESCRIBING PHYSICIAN				
RESULT & COMMENTS				

MEDICATION NAME	DATE STARTED	START DOSE	DATE ENDED	END DOSE
FREQUENCY				
PRESCRIBING PHYSICIAN				
RESULT & COMMENTS				

TREATMENT HISTORY - MEDICATION

MEDICATION NAME	DATE STARTED	START DOSE	DATE ENDED	END DOSE
FREQUENCY				
PRESCRIBING PHYSICIAN				
RESULT & COMMENTS				

MEDICATION NAME	DATE STARTED	START DOSE	DATE ENDED	END DOSE
FREQUENCY				
PRESCRIBING PHYSICIAN				
RESULT & COMMENTS				

MEDICATION NAME	DATE STARTED	START DOSE	DATE ENDED	END DOSE
FREQUENCY				
PRESCRIBING PHYSICIAN				
RESULT & COMMENTS				

TREATMENT HISTORY - MEDICATION

MEDICATION NAME	DATE STARTED	START DOSE	DATE ENDED	END DOSE
FREQUENCY				
PRESCRIBING PHYSICIAN				
RESULT & COMMENTS				

MEDICATION NAME	DATE STARTED	START DOSE	DATE ENDED	END DOSE
FREQUENCY				
PRESCRIBING PHYSICIAN				
RESULT & COMMENTS				

MEDICATION NAME	DATE STARTED	START DOSE	DATE ENDED	END DOSE
FREQUENCY				
PRESCRIBING PHYSICIAN				
RESULT & COMMENTS				

TREATMENT HISTORY - MEDICATION

MEDICATION NAME	DATE STARTED	START DOSE	DATE ENDED	END DOSE
FREQUENCY				
PRESCRIBING PHYSICIAN				
RESULT & COMMENTS				

MEDICATION NAME	DATE STARTED	START DOSE	DATE ENDED	END DOSE
FREQUENCY				
PRESCRIBING PHYSICIAN				
RESULT & COMMENTS				

MEDICATION NAME	DATE STARTED	START DOSE	DATE ENDED	END DOSE
FREQUENCY				
PRESCRIBING PHYSICIAN				
RESULT & COMMENTS				

TREATMENT HISTORY - MEDICATION

MEDICATION NAME	DATE STARTED	START DOSE	DATE ENDED	END DOSE
FREQUENCY				
PRESCRIBING PHYSICIAN				
RESULT & COMMENTS				

MEDICATION NAME	DATE STARTED	START DOSE	DATE ENDED	END DOSE
FREQUENCY				
PRESCRIBING PHYSICIAN				
RESULT & COMMENTS				

MEDICATION NAME	DATE STARTED	START DOSE	DATE ENDED	END DOSE
FREQUENCY				
PRESCRIBING PHYSICIAN				
RESULT & COMMENTS				

TREATMENT HISTORY - MEDICATION

MEDICATION NAME	DATE STARTED	START DOSE	DATE ENDED	END DOSE
FREQUENCY				
PRESCRIBING PHYSICIAN				
RESULT & COMMENTS				

MEDICATION NAME	DATE STARTED	START DOSE	DATE ENDED	END DOSE
FREQUENCY				
PRESCRIBING PHYSICIAN				
RESULT & COMMENTS				

MEDICATION NAME	DATE STARTED	START DOSE	DATE ENDED	END DOSE
FREQUENCY				
PRESCRIBING PHYSICIAN				
RESULT & COMMENTS				

TREATMENT HISTORY - MEDICATION

MEDICATION NAME	DATE STARTED	START DOSE	DATE ENDED	END DOSE
FREQUENCY				
PRESCRIBING PHYSICIAN				
RESULT & COMMENTS				

MEDICATION NAME	DATE STARTED	START DOSE	DATE ENDED	END DOSE
FREQUENCY				
PRESCRIBING PHYSICIAN				
RESULT & COMMENTS				

MEDICATION NAME	DATE STARTED	START DOSE	DATE ENDED	END DOSE
FREQUENCY				
PRESCRIBING PHYSICIAN				
RESULT & COMMENTS				

TREATMENT HISTORY - MEDICATION

MEDICATION NAME	DATE STARTED	START DOSE	DATE ENDED	END DOSE
FREQUENCY				
PRESCRIBING PHYSICIAN				
RESULT & COMMENTS				

MEDICATION NAME	DATE STARTED	START DOSE	DATE ENDED	END DOSE
FREQUENCY				
PRESCRIBING PHYSICIAN				
RESULT & COMMENTS				

MEDICATION NAME	DATE STARTED	START DOSE	DATE ENDED	END DOSE
FREQUENCY				
PRESCRIBING PHYSICIAN				
RESULT & COMMENTS				

TREATMENT HISTORY - MEDICATION

MEDICATION NAME	DATE STARTED	START DOSE	DATE ENDED	END DOSE
FREQUENCY				
PRESCRIBING PHYSICIAN				
RESULT & COMMENTS				

MEDICATION NAME	DATE STARTED	START DOSE	DATE ENDED	END DOSE
FREQUENCY				
PRESCRIBING PHYSICIAN				
RESULT & COMMENTS				

MEDICATION NAME	DATE STARTED	START DOSE	DATE ENDED	END DOSE
FREQUENCY				
PRESCRIBING PHYSICIAN				
RESULT & COMMENTS				

TREATMENT HISTORY - MEDICATION

MEDICATION NAME	DATE STARTED	START DOSE	DATE ENDED	END DOSE
FREQUENCY				
PRESCRIBING PHYSICIAN				
RESULT & COMMENTS				

MEDICATION NAME	DATE STARTED	START DOSE	DATE ENDED	END DOSE
FREQUENCY				
PRESCRIBING PHYSICIAN				
RESULT & COMMENTS				

MEDICATION NAME	DATE STARTED	START DOSE	DATE ENDED	END DOSE
FREQUENCY				
PRESCRIBING PHYSICIAN				
RESULT & COMMENTS				

TREATMENT HISTORY - MEDICATION

MEDICATION NAME	DATE STARTED	START DOSE	DATE ENDED	END DOSE
FREQUENCY				
PRESCRIBING PHYSICIAN				
RESULT & COMMENTS				

MEDICATION NAME	DATE STARTED	START DOSE	DATE ENDED	END DOSE
FREQUENCY				
PRESCRIBING PHYSICIAN				
RESULT & COMMENTS				

MEDICATION NAME	DATE STARTED	START DOSE	DATE ENDED	END DOSE
FREQUENCY				
PRESCRIBING PHYSICIAN				
RESULT & COMMENTS				

TREATMENT HISTORY - MEDICATION

MEDICATION NAME	DATE STARTED	START DOSE	DATE ENDED	END DOSE
FREQUENCY				
PRESCRIBING PHYSICIAN				
RESULT & COMMENTS				

MEDICATION NAME	DATE STARTED	START DOSE	DATE ENDED	END DOSE
FREQUENCY				
PRESCRIBING PHYSICIAN				
RESULT & COMMENTS				

MEDICATION NAME	DATE STARTED	START DOSE	DATE ENDED	END DOSE
FREQUENCY				
PRESCRIBING PHYSICIAN				
RESULT & COMMENTS				

TREATMENT HISTORY - MEDICATION

MEDICATION NAME	DATE STARTED	START DOSE	DATE ENDED	END DOSE
FREQUENCY				
PRESCRIBING PHYSICIAN				
RESULT & COMMENTS				

MEDICATION NAME	DATE STARTED	START DOSE	DATE ENDED	END DOSE
FREQUENCY				
PRESCRIBING PHYSICIAN				
RESULT & COMMENTS				

MEDICATION NAME	DATE STARTED	START DOSE	DATE ENDED	END DOSE
FREQUENCY				
PRESCRIBING PHYSICIAN				
RESULT & COMMENTS				

TREATMENT HISTORY - MEDICATION

MEDICATION NAME	DATE STARTED	START DOSE	DATE ENDED	END DOSE
FREQUENCY				
PRESCRIBING PHYSICIAN				
RESULT & COMMENTS				

MEDICATION NAME	DATE STARTED	START DOSE	DATE ENDED	END DOSE
FREQUENCY				
PRESCRIBING PHYSICIAN				
RESULT & COMMENTS				

MEDICATION NAME	DATE STARTED	START DOSE	DATE ENDED	END DOSE
FREQUENCY				
PRESCRIBING PHYSICIAN				
RESULT & COMMENTS				

TREATMENT HISTORY - MEDICATION

MEDICATION NAME	DATE STARTED	START DOSE	DATE ENDED	END DOSE
FREQUENCY				
PRESCRIBING PHYSICIAN				
RESULT & COMMENTS				

MEDICATION NAME	DATE STARTED	START DOSE	DATE ENDED	END DOSE
FREQUENCY				
PRESCRIBING PHYSICIAN				
RESULT & COMMENTS				

MEDICATION NAME	DATE STARTED	START DOSE	DATE ENDED	END DOSE
FREQUENCY				
PRESCRIBING PHYSICIAN				
RESULT & COMMENTS				

TREATMENT HISTORY - MEDICATION

MEDICATION NAME	DATE STARTED	START DOSE	DATE ENDED	END DOSE
FREQUENCY				
PRESCRIBING PHYSICIAN				
RESULT & COMMENTS				

MEDICATION NAME	DATE STARTED	START DOSE	DATE ENDED	END DOSE
FREQUENCY				
PRESCRIBING PHYSICIAN				
RESULT & COMMENTS				

MEDICATION NAME	DATE STARTED	START DOSE	DATE ENDED	END DOSE
FREQUENCY				
PRESCRIBING PHYSICIAN				
RESULT & COMMENTS				

TREATMENT HISTORY - MEDICATION

MEDICATION NAME	DATE STARTED	START DOSE	DATE ENDED	END DOSE
FREQUENCY				
PRESCRIBING PHYSICIAN				
RESULT & COMMENTS				

MEDICATION NAME	DATE STARTED	START DOSE	DATE ENDED	END DOSE
FREQUENCY				
PRESCRIBING PHYSICIAN				
RESULT & COMMENTS				

MEDICATION NAME	DATE STARTED	START DOSE	DATE ENDED	END DOSE
FREQUENCY				
PRESCRIBING PHYSICIAN				
RESULT & COMMENTS				

SYMPTOM - TRACKER

DATE & TIME _____

DESCRIPTION
_____

BODY TEMPERATURE

OBSERVATIONS
_____
_____

PHYSICAL SYMPTOMS	FEVER		SNEEZING		RASH		Other	
POSSIBLE TRIGGERS	FOOD		WEATHER		MEDICATION		Other	

ACTION TAKEN _____
_____

SYMPTOM - TRACKER

DATE & TIME _____

DESCRIPTION
_____

BODY TEMPERATURE

OBSERVATIONS
_____
_____

PHYSICAL SYMPTOMS	FEVER		SNEEZING		RASH		Other	
POSSIBLE TRIGGERS	FOOD		WEATHER		MEDICATION		Other	

ACTION TAKEN _____
_____

SYMPTOM - TRACKER

DATE & TIME_____

DESCRIPTION
_____

BODY TEMPERATURE

OBSERVATIONS
_____
_____

PHYSICAL SYMPTOMS	FEVER		SNEEZING		RASH		Other	
POSSIBLE TRIGGERS	FOOD		WEATHER		MEDICATION		Other	

ACTION TAKEN_____
_____

SYMPTOM - TRACKER

DATE & TIME_____

DESCRIPTION
_____

BODY TEMPERATURE

OBSERVATIONS
_____
_____

PHYSICAL SYMPTOMS	FEVER		SNEEZING		RASH		Other	
POSSIBLE TRIGGERS	FOOD		WEATHER		MEDICATION		Other	

ACTION TAKEN_____
_____

SYMPTOM - TRACKER

DATE & TIME _____

DESCRIPTION
_____

BODY TEMPERATURE _____

OBSERVATIONS
_____
_____

PHYSICAL SYMPTOMS	FEVER		SNEEZING		RASH		Other	
POSSIBLE TRIGGERS	FOOD		WEATHER		MEDICATION		Other	

ACTION TAKEN _____
_____

SYMPTOM - TRACKER

DATE & TIME _____

DESCRIPTION
_____

BODY TEMPERATURE _____

OBSERVATIONS
_____
_____

PHYSICAL SYMPTOMS	FEVER		SNEEZING		RASH		Other	
POSSIBLE TRIGGERS	FOOD		WEATHER		MEDICATION		Other	

ACTION TAKEN _____
_____

SYMPTOM - TRACKER

DATE & TIME _____

DESCRIPTION
_____

BODY TEMPERATURE

OBSERVATIONS
_____
_____

PHYSICAL SYMPTOMS	FEVER		SNEEZING		RASH		Other	
POSSIBLE TRIGGERS	FOOD		WEATHER		MEDICATION		Other	

ACTION TAKEN _____
_____

SYMPTOM - TRACKER

DATE & TIME _____

DESCRIPTION
_____

BODY TEMPERATURE

OBSERVATIONS
_____
_____

PHYSICAL SYMPTOMS	FEVER		SNEEZING		RASH		Other	
POSSIBLE TRIGGERS	FOOD		WEATHER		MEDICATION		Other	

ACTION TAKEN _____
_____

SYMPTOM - TRACKER

DATE & TIME _____

DESCRIPTION
_____

BODY TEMPERATURE

OBSERVATIONS
_____
_____

PHYSICAL SYMPTOMS	FEVER		SNEEZING		RASH		Other	
POSSIBLE TRIGGERS	FOOD		WEATHER		MEDICATION		Other	

ACTION TAKEN _____
_____

SYMPTOM - TRACKER

DATE & TIME _____

DESCRIPTION
_____

BODY TEMPERATURE

OBSERVATIONS
_____
_____

PHYSICAL SYMPTOMS	FEVER		SNEEZING		RASH		Other	
POSSIBLE TRIGGERS	FOOD		WEATHER		MEDICATION		Other	

ACTION TAKEN _____
_____

SYMPTOM - TRACKER

DATE & TIME _____

DESCRIPTION
_____

BODY TEMPERATURE

OBSERVATIONS
_____
_____

PHYSICAL SYMPTOMS	FEVER		SNEEZING		RASH		Other	
POSSIBLE TRIGGERS	FOOD		WEATHER		MEDICATION		Other	

ACTION TAKEN _____
_____

SYMPTOM - TRACKER

DATE & TIME _____

DESCRIPTION
_____

BODY TEMPERATURE

OBSERVATIONS
_____
_____

PHYSICAL SYMPTOMS	FEVER		SNEEZING		RASH		Other	
POSSIBLE TRIGGERS	FOOD		WEATHER		MEDICATION		Other	

ACTION TAKEN _____
_____

SYMPTOM - TRACKER

DATE & TIME _____

DESCRIPTION
_____

BODY TEMPERATURE

OBSERVATIONS
_____
_____

PHYSICAL SYMPTOMS	FEVER		SNEEZING		RASH		Other	
POSSIBLE TRIGGERS	FOOD		WEATHER		MEDICATION		Other	

ACTION TAKEN _____
_____

SYMPTOM - TRACKER

DATE & TIME _____

DESCRIPTION
_____

BODY TEMPERATURE

OBSERVATIONS
_____
_____

PHYSICAL SYMPTOMS	FEVER		SNEEZING		RASH		Other	
POSSIBLE TRIGGERS	FOOD		WEATHER		MEDICATION		Other	

ACTION TAKEN _____
_____

SYMPTOM - TRACKER

DATE & TIME _____

DESCRIPTION
_____

BODY TEMPERATURE
_____

OBSERVATIONS
_____
_____

PHYSICAL SYMPTOMS	FEVER		SNEEZING		RASH		Other	
POSSIBLE TRIGGERS	FOOD		WEATHER		MEDICATION		Other	

ACTION TAKEN _____
_____

SYMPTOM - TRACKER

DATE & TIME _____

DESCRIPTION
_____

BODY TEMPERATURE
_____

OBSERVATIONS
_____
_____

PHYSICAL SYMPTOMS	FEVER		SNEEZING		RASH		Other	
POSSIBLE TRIGGERS	FOOD		WEATHER		MEDICATION		Other	

ACTION TAKEN _____
_____

SYMPTOM - TRACKER

DATE & TIME _____

DESCRIPTION
_____

BODY TEMPERATURE
_____

OBSERVATIONS
_____
_____

PHYSICAL SYMPTOMS	FEVER		SNEEZING		RASH		Other	
POSSIBLE TRIGGERS	FOOD		WEATHER		MEDICATION		Other	

ACTION TAKEN _____
_____

SYMPTOM - TRACKER

DATE & TIME _____

DESCRIPTION
_____

BODY TEMPERATURE
_____

OBSERVATIONS
_____
_____

PHYSICAL SYMPTOMS	FEVER		SNEEZING		RASH		Other	
POSSIBLE TRIGGERS	FOOD		WEATHER		MEDICATION		Other	

ACTION TAKEN _____
_____

SYMPTOM - TRACKER

DATE & TIME _____

DESCRIPTION
_____

BODY TEMPERATURE

OBSERVATIONS
_____
_____

PHYSICAL SYMPTOMS	FEVER		SNEEZING		RASH		Other	
POSSIBLE TRIGGERS	FOOD		WEATHER		MEDICATION		Other	

ACTION TAKEN _____
_____

SYMPTOM - TRACKER

DATE & TIME _____

DESCRIPTION
_____

BODY TEMPERATURE

OBSERVATIONS
_____
_____

PHYSICAL SYMPTOMS	FEVER		SNEEZING		RASH		Other	
POSSIBLE TRIGGERS	FOOD		WEATHER		MEDICATION		Other	

ACTION TAKEN _____
_____

SYMPTOM - TRACKER

DATE & TIME _____

DESCRIPTION
_____

BODY TEMPERATURE _____

OBSERVATIONS
_____
_____

PHYSICAL SYMPTOMS	FEVER		SNEEZING		RASH		Other	
POSSIBLE TRIGGERS	FOOD		WEATHER		MEDICATION		Other	

ACTION TAKEN _____
_____

SYMPTOM - TRACKER

DATE & TIME _____

DESCRIPTION
_____

BODY TEMPERATURE _____

OBSERVATIONS
_____
_____

PHYSICAL SYMPTOMS	FEVER		SNEEZING		RASH		Other	
POSSIBLE TRIGGERS	FOOD		WEATHER		MEDICATION		Other	

ACTION TAKEN _____
_____

SYMPTOM - TRACKER

DATE & TIME _____

DESCRIPTION
_____

BODY TEMPERATURE
_____

OBSERVATIONS
_____
_____

PHYSICAL SYMPTOMS	FEVER		SNEEZING		RASH		Other	
POSSIBLE TRIGGERS	FOOD		WEATHER		MEDICATION		Other	

ACTION TAKEN _____
_____

SYMPTOM - TRACKER

DATE & TIME _____

DESCRIPTION
_____

BODY TEMPERATURE
_____

OBSERVATIONS
_____
_____

PHYSICAL SYMPTOMS	FEVER		SNEEZING		RASH		Other	
POSSIBLE TRIGGERS	FOOD		WEATHER		MEDICATION		Other	

ACTION TAKEN _____
_____

SYMPTOM - TRACKER

DATE & TIME_____

DESCRIPTION
_____

BODY TEMPERATURE

OBSERVATIONS
_____
_____

PHYSICAL SYMPTOMS	FEVER		SNEEZING		RASH		Other	
POSSIBLE TRIGGERS	FOOD		WEATHER		MEDICATION		Other	

ACTION TAKEN_____
_____

SYMPTOM - TRACKER

DATE & TIME_____

DESCRIPTION
_____

BODY TEMPERATURE

OBSERVATIONS
_____
_____

PHYSICAL SYMPTOMS	FEVER		SNEEZING		RASH		Other	
POSSIBLE TRIGGERS	FOOD		WEATHER		MEDICATION		Other	

ACTION TAKEN_____
_____

SYMPTOM - TRACKER

DATE & TIME _____

DESCRIPTION
_____

BODY TEMPERATURE
_____

OBSERVATIONS
_____
_____

PHYSICAL SYMPTOMS	FEVER		SNEEZING		RASH		Other	
POSSIBLE TRIGGERS	FOOD		WEATHER		MEDICATION		Other	

ACTION TAKEN _____
_____

SYMPTOM - TRACKER

DATE & TIME _____

DESCRIPTION
_____

BODY TEMPERATURE
_____

OBSERVATIONS
_____
_____

PHYSICAL SYMPTOMS	FEVER		SNEEZING		RASH		Other	
POSSIBLE TRIGGERS	FOOD		WEATHER		MEDICATION		Other	

ACTION TAKEN _____
_____

SYMPTOM - TRACKER

DATE & TIME _____

DESCRIPTION
_____

BODY TEMPERATURE

OBSERVATIONS
_____
_____

PHYSICAL SYMPTOMS	FEVER		SNEEZING		RASH		Other	
POSSIBLE TRIGGERS	FOOD		WEATHER		MEDICATION		Other	

ACTION TAKEN _____
_____

SYMPTOM - TRACKER

DATE & TIME _____

DESCRIPTION
_____

BODY TEMPERATURE

OBSERVATIONS
_____
_____

PHYSICAL SYMPTOMS	FEVER		SNEEZING		RASH		Other	
POSSIBLE TRIGGERS	FOOD		WEATHER		MEDICATION		Other	

ACTION TAKEN _____
_____

SYMPTOM - TRACKER

DATE & TIME _____

DESCRIPTION
_____

BODY TEMPERATURE _____

OBSERVATIONS
_____
_____

PHYSICAL SYMPTOMS	FEVER		SNEEZING		RASH		Other	
POSSIBLE TRIGGERS	FOOD		WEATHER		MEDICATION		Other	

ACTION TAKEN _____
_____

SYMPTOM - TRACKER

DATE & TIME _____

DESCRIPTION
_____

BODY TEMPERATURE _____

OBSERVATIONS
_____
_____

PHYSICAL SYMPTOMS	FEVER		SNEEZING		RASH		Other	
POSSIBLE TRIGGERS	FOOD		WEATHER		MEDICATION		Other	

ACTION TAKEN _____
_____

SYMPTOM - TRACKER

DATE & TIME _____

DESCRIPTION
_____

BODY TEMPERATURE

OBSERVATIONS
_____
_____

PHYSICAL SYMPTOMS	FEVER		SNEEZING		RASH		Other	
POSSIBLE TRIGGERS	FOOD		WEATHER		MEDICATION		Other	

ACTION TAKEN _____
_____

SYMPTOM - TRACKER

DATE & TIME _____

DESCRIPTION
_____

BODY TEMPERATURE

OBSERVATIONS
_____
_____

PHYSICAL SYMPTOMS	FEVER		SNEEZING		RASH		Other	
POSSIBLE TRIGGERS	FOOD		WEATHER		MEDICATION		Other	

ACTION TAKEN _____
_____

SYMPTOM - TRACKER

DATE & TIME _____

DESCRIPTION
_____

BODY TEMPERATURE

OBSERVATIONS
_____
_____

PHYSICAL SYMPTOMS	FEVER		SNEEZING		RASH		Other	
POSSIBLE TRIGGERS	FOOD		WEATHER		MEDICATION		Other	

ACTION TAKEN _____
_____

SYMPTOM - TRACKER

DATE & TIME _____

DESCRIPTION
_____

BODY TEMPERATURE

OBSERVATIONS
_____
_____

PHYSICAL SYMPTOMS	FEVER		SNEEZING		RASH		Other	
POSSIBLE TRIGGERS	FOOD		WEATHER		MEDICATION		Other	

ACTION TAKEN _____
_____

SYMPTOM - TRACKER

DATE & TIME _____

DESCRIPTION
_____

BODY TEMPERATURE

OBSERVATIONS
_____
_____

PHYSICAL SYMPTOMS	FEVER		SNEEZING		RASH		Other	
POSSIBLE TRIGGERS	FOOD		WEATHER		MEDICATION		Other	

ACTION TAKEN _____
_____

SYMPTOM - TRACKER

DATE & TIME _____

DESCRIPTION
_____

BODY TEMPERATURE

OBSERVATIONS
_____
_____

PHYSICAL SYMPTOMS	FEVER		SNEEZING		RASH		Other	
POSSIBLE TRIGGERS	FOOD		WEATHER		MEDICATION		Other	

ACTION TAKEN _____
_____

SYMPTOM - TRACKER

DATE & TIME _____

DESCRIPTION
_____

BODY TEMPERATURE

OBSERVATIONS
_____
_____

PHYSICAL SYMPTOMS	FEVER		SNEEZING		RASH		Other	
POSSIBLE TRIGGERS	FOOD		WEATHER		MEDICATION		Other	

ACTION TAKEN _____
_____

SYMPTOM - TRACKER

DATE & TIME _____

DESCRIPTION
_____

BODY TEMPERATURE

OBSERVATIONS
_____
_____

PHYSICAL SYMPTOMS	FEVER		SNEEZING		RASH		Other	
POSSIBLE TRIGGERS	FOOD		WEATHER		MEDICATION		Other	

ACTION TAKEN _____
_____

TREATMENT HISTORY - VISITS

DATE	TIME	LOCATION
REASON FOR VISIT		
TEST		
RESULT		
DIAGNOSIS		
TREATMENT		
COMMENTS		

DATE	TIME	LOCATION
REASON FOR VISIT		
TEST		
RESULT		
DIAGNOSIS		
TREATMENT		
COMMENTS		

TREATMENT HISTORY - VISITS

DATE	TIME	LOCATION
REASON FOR VISIT		

TEST	
RESULT	
DIAGNOSIS	
TREATMENT	
COMMENTS	

DATE	TIME	LOCATION
REASON FOR VISIT		

TEST	
RESULT	
DIAGNOSIS	
TREATMENT	
COMMENTS	

TREATMENT HISTORY - VISITS

DATE	TIME	LOCATION
REASON FOR VISIT		
TEST		
RESULT		
DIAGNOSIS		
TREATMENT		
COMMENTS		

DATE	TIME	LOCATION
REASON FOR VISIT		
TEST		
RESULT		
DIAGNOSIS		
TREATMENT		
COMMENTS		

TREATMENT HISTORY - VISITS

DATE	TIME	LOCATION

REASON FOR VISIT	

TEST	
RESULT	
DIAGNOSIS	
TREATMENT	
COMMENTS	

DATE	TIME	LOCATION

REASON FOR VISIT	

TEST	
RESULT	
DIAGNOSIS	
TREATMENT	
COMMENTS	

TREATMENT HISTORY - VISITS

DATE	TIME	LOCATION

REASON FOR VISIT	

TEST	
RESULT	
DIAGNOSIS	
TREATMENT	
COMMENTS	

DATE	TIME	LOCATION

REASON FOR VISIT	

TEST	
RESULT	
DIAGNOSIS	
TREATMENT	
COMMENTS	

TREATMENT HISTORY - VISITS

DATE	TIME	LOCATION

REASON FOR VISIT	

TEST	
RESULT	
DIAGNOSIS	
TREATMENT	
COMMENTS	

DATE	TIME	LOCATION

REASON FOR VISIT	

TEST	
RESULT	
DIAGNOSIS	
TREATMENT	
COMMENTS	

TREATMENT HISTORY - VISITS

DATE	TIME	LOCATION
REASON FOR VISIT		
TEST		
RESULT		
DIAGNOSIS		
TREATMENT		
COMMENTS		

DATE	TIME	LOCATION
REASON FOR VISIT		
TEST		
RESULT		
DIAGNOSIS		
TREATMENT		
COMMENTS		

TREATMENT HISTORY - VISITS

DATE	TIME	LOCATION

REASON FOR VISIT	

TEST	
RESULT	
DIAGNOSIS	
TREATMENT	
COMMENTS	

DATE	TIME	LOCATION

REASON FOR VISIT	

TEST	
RESULT	
DIAGNOSIS	
TREATMENT	
COMMENTS	

TREATMENT HISTORY - VISITS

DATE	TIME	LOCATION

REASON FOR VISIT	

TEST	
RESULT	
DIAGNOSIS	
TREATMENT	
COMMENTS	

DATE	TIME	LOCATION

REASON FOR VISIT	

TEST	
RESULT	
DIAGNOSIS	
TREATMENT	
COMMENTS	

TREATMENT HISTORY - VISITS

DATE	TIME	LOCATION

REASON FOR VISIT	

TEST	
RESULT	
DIAGNOSIS	
TREATMENT	
COMMENTS	

DATE	TIME	LOCATION

REASON FOR VISIT	

TEST	
RESULT	
DIAGNOSIS	
TREATMENT	
COMMENTS	

TREATMENT HISTORY - VISITS

DATE	TIME	LOCATION
REASON FOR VISIT		
TEST		
RESULT		
DIAGNOSIS		
TREATMENT		
COMMENTS		

DATE	TIME	LOCATION
REASON FOR VISIT		
TEST		
RESULT		
DIAGNOSIS		
TREATMENT		
COMMENTS		

TREATMENT HISTORY - VISITS

DATE	TIME	LOCATION

REASON FOR VISIT	

TEST	
RESULT	
DIAGNOSIS	
TREATMENT	
COMMENTS	

DATE	TIME	LOCATION

REASON FOR VISIT	

TEST	
RESULT	
DIAGNOSIS	
TREATMENT	
COMMENTS	

TREATMENT HISTORY - VISITS

DATE	TIME	LOCATION

REASON FOR VISIT	

TEST	
RESULT	
DIAGNOSIS	
TREATMENT	
COMMENTS	

DATE	TIME	LOCATION

REASON FOR VISIT	

TEST	
RESULT	
DIAGNOSIS	
TREATMENT	
COMMENTS	

TREATMENT HISTORY - VISITS

DATE	TIME	LOCATION
REASON FOR VISIT		
TEST		
RESULT		
DIAGNOSIS		
TREATMENT		
COMMENTS		

DATE	TIME	LOCATION
REASON FOR VISIT		
TEST		
RESULT		
DIAGNOSIS		
TREATMENT		
COMMENTS		

TREATMENT HISTORY - VISITS

DATE	TIME	LOCATION
REASON FOR VISIT		
TEST		
RESULT		
DIAGNOSIS		
TREATMENT		
COMMENTS		

DATE	TIME	LOCATION
REASON FOR VISIT		
TEST		
RESULT		
DIAGNOSIS		
TREATMENT		
COMMENTS		

TREATMENT HISTORY - VISITS

DATE	TIME	LOCATION
REASON FOR VISIT		
TEST		
RESULT		
DIAGNOSIS		
TREATMENT		
COMMENTS		

DATE	TIME	LOCATION
REASON FOR VISIT		
TEST		
RESULT		
DIAGNOSIS		
TREATMENT		
COMMENTS		

TREATMENT HISTORY - VISITS

DATE	TIME	LOCATION
REASON FOR VISIT		
TEST		
RESULT		
DIAGNOSIS		
TREATMENT		
COMMENTS		

DATE	TIME	LOCATION
REASON FOR VISIT		
TEST		
RESULT		
DIAGNOSIS		
TREATMENT		
COMMENTS		

TREATMENT HISTORY - VISITS

DATE	TIME	LOCATION
REASON FOR VISIT		

TEST	
RESULT	
DIAGNOSIS	
TREATMENT	
COMMENTS	

DATE	TIME	LOCATION
REASON FOR VISIT		

TEST	
RESULT	
DIAGNOSIS	
TREATMENT	
COMMENTS	

TREATMENT HISTORY - VISITS

DATE	TIME	LOCATION
REASON FOR VISIT		
TEST		
RESULT		
DIAGNOSIS		
TREATMENT		
COMMENTS		

DATE	TIME	LOCATION
REASON FOR VISIT		
TEST		
RESULT		
DIAGNOSIS		
TREATMENT		
COMMENTS		

TREATMENT HISTORY - VISITS

DATE	TIME	LOCATION

REASON FOR VISIT	

TEST	
RESULT	
DIAGNOSIS	
TREATMENT	
COMMENTS	

DATE	TIME	LOCATION

REASON FOR VISIT	

TEST	
RESULT	
DIAGNOSIS	
TREATMENT	
COMMENTS	

TREATMENT HISTORY - VISITS

DATE	TIME	LOCATION

REASON FOR VISIT	

TEST	
RESULT	
DIAGNOSIS	
TREATMENT	
COMMENTS	

DATE	TIME	LOCATION

REASON FOR VISIT	

TEST	
RESULT	
DIAGNOSIS	
TREATMENT	
COMMENTS	

TREATMENT HISTORY - VISITS

DATE	TIME	LOCATION

REASON FOR VISIT	

TEST	
RESULT	
DIAGNOSIS	
TREATMENT	
COMMENTS	

DATE	TIME	LOCATION

REASON FOR VISIT	

TEST	
RESULT	
DIAGNOSIS	
TREATMENT	
COMMENTS	

TREATMENT HISTORY - VISITS

DATE	TIME	LOCATION

REASON FOR VISIT	

TEST	
RESULT	
DIAGNOSIS	
TREATMENT	
COMMENTS	

DATE	TIME	LOCATION

REASON FOR VISIT	

TEST	
RESULT	
DIAGNOSIS	
TREATMENT	
COMMENTS	

TREATMENT HISTORY - VISITS

DATE	TIME	LOCATION

REASON FOR VISIT	

TEST	
RESULT	
DIAGNOSIS	
TREATMENT	
COMMENTS	

DATE	TIME	LOCATION

REASON FOR VISIT	

TEST	
RESULT	
DIAGNOSIS	
TREATMENT	
COMMENTS	

TREATMENT HISTORY - VISITS

DATE	TIME	LOCATION
REASON FOR VISIT		
TEST		
RESULT		
DIAGNOSIS		
TREATMENT		
COMMENTS		

DATE	TIME	LOCATION
REASON FOR VISIT		
TEST		
RESULT		
DIAGNOSIS		
TREATMENT		
COMMENTS		

GROWTH LOG

DATE	AGE	HEIGHT

WEIGHT LOG

DATE	AGE	WEIGHT

GROWTH LOG

DATE	AGE	HEIGHT

WEIGHT LOG

DATE	AGE	WEIGHT

TOOTH CHART

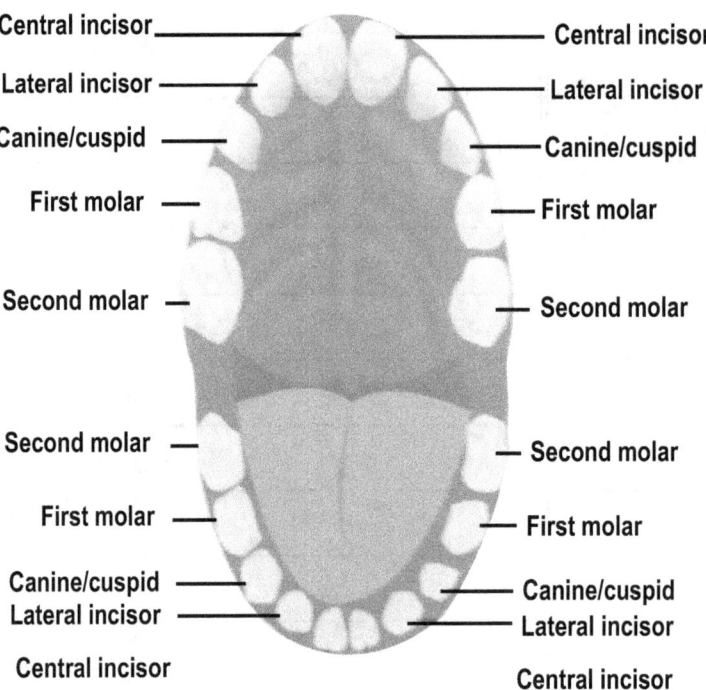

TOOTH RECORD - ADULT TEETH

TOOTH LOCATION	DATE

NOTES

NOTES

NOTES

NOTES

NOTES

NOTES

NOTES

NOTES

NOTES

NOTES

www.ingramcontent.com/pod-product-compliance
Lightning Source LLC
Chambersburg PA
CBHW081442220526
45466CB00008B/2483